THE 100 DIET JOURNAL
The Handy Companion to Track Your Progress on The 100 Diet

ISBN-13:978-1506090306
ISBN-10:1506090303

©2014 My Personal Journals
www.remarkableauthor.com/mpj

Free Gift for You

To get your free copy of

"How to Stay Motivated
and Lose Weight"

visit

www.staymotivatedclub.com/100

MEASURING YOUR SUCCESS

Progress Chart

	Weight	Loss	Overall Quiz Results
Week 1			
Week 2			
Week 3			
Week 4			
Week 5			
Week 6			
Week 7			
Week 8			
Week 9			
Week 10			
Total Loss			

Body Measurements Chart

Measurement	Week 1	Week 3	Week 5	Week 7	Week 9	Inches Lost
Bust						
Chest						
Waist						
Hips						
Thigh						
Calves						
Upper arm						
Forearm						

BEFORE PICTURE

MY WEIGHT_____

WHAT I'M THINKING/HOW I FEEL: _____

_____

_____

_____

_____

_____

_____

RULES TO FOLLOW

RULES TO FOLLOW

WEEKLY MEAL PLANNER
Week of _____

	BREAKFAST	LUNCH	DINNER	SNACKS
MON				
TUE				
WED				
THU				
FRI				
SAT				
SUN				

DAY 1 – Date_____

	FOOD ITEM	TOTAL SUGAR CALORIES
MEAL 1		
SNACK		
MEAL 2		
SNACK		
MEAL 3		
SNACK		
	TOTAL:	

NOTES/ACCOMPLISHMENTS

_____
_____
_____

DAY 2 – Date_____

	FOOD ITEM	TOTAL SUGAR CALORIES
MEAL 1		
SNACK		
MEAL 2		
SNACK		
MEAL 3		
SNACK		
	TOTAL:	

NOTES/ACCOMPLISHMENTS

_____

_____

_____

DAY 3 – Date_____

	FOOD ITEM	TOTAL SUGAR CALORIES
MEAL 1		
SNACK		
MEAL 2		
SNACK		
MEAL 3		
SNACK		
	TOTAL:	

NOTES/ACCOMPLISHMENTS

DAY 4 – Date_____

	FOOD ITEM	TOTAL SUGAR CALORIES
MEAL 1		
SNACK		
MEAL 2		
SNACK		
MEAL 3		
SNACK		
	TOTAL:	

NOTES/ACCOMPLISHMENTS

_____
_____
_____

DAY 5 – Date_____

	FOOD ITEM	TOTAL SUGAR CALORIES
MEAL 1		
SNACK		
MEAL 2		
SNACK		
MEAL 3		
SNACK		
	TOTAL:	

NOTES/ACCOMPLISHMENTS

DAY 6 – Date_____

	FOOD ITEM	TOTAL SUGAR CALORIES
MEAL 1		
SNACK		
MEAL 2		
SNACK		
MEAL 3		
SNACK		
	TOTAL:	

NOTES/ACCOMPLISHMENTS

DAY 7 – Date_____

	FOOD ITEM	TOTAL SUGAR CALORIES
MEAL 1		
SNACK		
MEAL 2		
SNACK		
MEAL 3		
SNACK		
	TOTAL:	

NOTES/ACCOMPLISHMENTS

WEEKLY MEAL PLANNER
Week of _____

	BREAKFAST	LUNCH	DINNER	SNACKS
MON				
TUE				
WED				
THU				
FRI				
SAT				
SUN				

DAY 8 – Date_____

	FOOD ITEM	TOTAL SUGAR CALORIES
MEAL 1		
SNACK		
MEAL 2		
SNACK		
MEAL 3		
SNACK		
	TOTAL:	

NOTES/ACCOMPLISHMENTS

DAY 9 – Date_____

	FOOD ITEM	TOTAL SUGAR CALORIES
MEAL 1		
SNACK		
MEAL 2		
SNACK		
MEAL 3		
SNACK		
	TOTAL:	

NOTES/ACCOMPLISHMENTS

DAY 10 – Date_____

	FOOD ITEM	TOTAL SUGAR CALORIES
MEAL 1		
SNACK		
MEAL 2		
SNACK		
MEAL 3		
SNACK		
	TOTAL:	

NOTES/ACCOMPLISHMENTS

DAY 11 – Date_____

	FOOD ITEM	TOTAL SUGAR CALORIES
MEAL 1		
SNACK		
MEAL 2		
SNACK		
MEAL 3		
SNACK		
	TOTAL:	

NOTES/ACCOMPLISHMENTS

DAY 12 – Date_____

	FOOD ITEM	TOTAL SUGAR CALORIES
MEAL 1		
SNACK		
MEAL 2		
SNACK		
MEAL 3		
SNACK		
	TOTAL:	

NOTES/ACCOMPLISHMENTS

DAY 13 – Date_____

	FOOD ITEM	TOTAL SUGAR CALORIES
MEAL 1		
SNACK		
MEAL 2		
SNACK		
MEAL 3		
SNACK		
	TOTAL:	

NOTES/ACCOMPLISHMENTS

DAY 14 – Date_____

	FOOD ITEM	TOTAL SUGAR CALORIES
MEAL 1		
SNACK		
MEAL 2		
SNACK		
MEAL 3		
SNACK		
	TOTAL:	

NOTES/ACCOMPLISHMENTS

WEEKLY MEAL PLANNER
Week of _____

	BREAKFAST	LUNCH	DINNER	SNACKS
MON				
TUE				
WED				
THU				
FRI				
SAT				
SUN				

DAY 15 – Date_____

	FOOD ITEM	TOTAL SUGAR CALORIES
MEAL 1		
SNACK		
MEAL 2		
SNACK		
MEAL 3		
SNACK		
	TOTAL:	

NOTES/ACCOMPLISHMENTS

DAY 16 – Date_____

	FOOD ITEM	TOTAL SUGAR CALORIES
MEAL 1		
SNACK		
MEAL 2		
SNACK		
MEAL 3		
SNACK		
	TOTAL:	

NOTES/ACCOMPLISHMENTS

DAY 17 – Date_____

	FOOD ITEM	TOTAL SUGAR CALORIES
MEAL 1		
SNACK		
MEAL 2		
SNACK		
MEAL 3		
SNACK		
	TOTAL:	

NOTES/ACCOMPLISHMENTS

DAY 18 – Date_____

	FOOD ITEM	TOTAL SUGAR CALORIES
MEAL 1		
SNACK		
MEAL 2		
SNACK		
MEAL 3		
SNACK		
	TOTAL:	

NOTES/ACCOMPLISHMENTS

DAY 19 – Date_____

	FOOD ITEM	TOTAL SUGAR CALORIES
MEAL 1		
SNACK		
MEAL 2		
SNACK		
MEAL 3		
SNACK		
	TOTAL:	

NOTES/ACCOMPLISHMENTS

DAY 20 – Date_____

	FOOD ITEM	TOTAL SUGAR CALORIES
MEAL 1		
SNACK		
MEAL 2		
SNACK		
MEAL 3		
SNACK		
	TOTAL:	

NOTES/ACCOMPLISHMENTS

DAY 21 – Date_____

	FOOD ITEM	TOTAL SUGAR CALORIES
MEAL 1		
SNACK		
MEAL 2		
SNACK		
MEAL 3		
SNACK		
	TOTAL:	

NOTES/ACCOMPLISHMENTS

WEEKLY MEAL PLANNER
Week of _____

	BREAKFAST	LUNCH	DINNER	SNACKS
MON				
TUE				
WED				
THU				
FRI				
SAT				
SUN				

DAY 22 – Date_____

	FOOD ITEM	TOTAL SUGAR CALORIES
MEAL 1		
SNACK		
MEAL 2		
SNACK		
MEAL 3		
SNACK		
	TOTAL:	

NOTES/ACCOMPLISHMENTS

DAY 23 – Date_____

	FOOD ITEM	TOTAL SUGAR CALORIES
MEAL 1		
SNACK		
MEAL 2		
SNACK		
MEAL 3		
SNACK		
	TOTAL:	

NOTES/ACCOMPLISHMENTS

DAY 24 – Date_____

	FOOD ITEM	TOTAL SUGAR CALORIES
MEAL 1		
SNACK		
MEAL 2		
SNACK		
MEAL 3		
SNACK		
	TOTAL:	

NOTES/ACCOMPLISHMENTS

DAY 25 – Date_____

	FOOD ITEM	TOTAL SUGAR CALORIES
MEAL 1		
SNACK		
MEAL 2		
SNACK		
MEAL 3		
SNACK		
	TOTAL:	

NOTES/ACCOMPLISHMENTS

DAY 26 – Date_____

	FOOD ITEM	TOTAL SUGAR CALORIES
MEAL 1		
SNACK		
MEAL 2		
SNACK		
MEAL 3		
SNACK		
	TOTAL:	

NOTES/ACCOMPLISHMENTS

DAY 27 – Date_____

	FOOD ITEM	TOTAL SUGAR CALORIES
MEAL 1		
SNACK		
MEAL 2		
SNACK		
MEAL 3		
SNACK		
	TOTAL:	

NOTES/ACCOMPLISHMENTS

DAY 28 – Date_____

	FOOD ITEM	TOTAL SUGAR CALORIES
MEAL 1		
SNACK		
MEAL 2		
SNACK		
MEAL 3		
SNACK		
	TOTAL:	

NOTES/ACCOMPLISHMENTS

WEEKLY MEAL PLANNER
Week of _____

	BREAKFAST	LUNCH	DINNER	SNACKS
MON				
TUE				
WED				
THU				
FRI				
SAT				
SUN				

DAY 29 – Date_____

	FOOD ITEM	TOTAL SUGAR CALORIES
MEAL 1		
SNACK		
MEAL 2		
SNACK		
MEAL 3		
SNACK		
	TOTAL:	

NOTES/ACCOMPLISHMENTS

DAY 30 – Date_____

	FOOD ITEM	TOTAL SUGAR CALORIES
MEAL 1		
SNACK		
MEAL 2		
SNACK		
MEAL 3		
SNACK		
	TOTAL:	

NOTES/ACCOMPLISHMENTS

MIDWAY PICTURE

MY WEIGHT_____

WHAT I'M THINKING/HOW I FEEL: _____

_____

_____

_____

_____

_____

_____

DAY 31 – Date_____

	FOOD ITEM	TOTAL SUGAR CALORIES
MEAL 1		
SNACK		
MEAL 2		
SNACK		
MEAL 3		
SNACK		
	TOTAL:	

NOTES/ACCOMPLISHMENTS

DAY 32 – Date_____

	FOOD ITEM	TOTAL SUGAR CALORIES
MEAL 1		
SNACK		
MEAL 2		
SNACK		
MEAL 3		
SNACK		
	TOTAL:	

NOTES/ACCOMPLISHMENTS

DAY 33 – Date_____

	FOOD ITEM	TOTAL SUGAR CALORIES
MEAL 1		
SNACK		
MEAL 2		
SNACK		
MEAL 3		
SNACK		
	TOTAL:	

NOTES/ACCOMPLISHMENTS

DAY 34 – Date_____

	FOOD ITEM	TOTAL SUGAR CALORIES
MEAL 1		
SNACK		
MEAL 2		
SNACK		
MEAL 3		
SNACK		
	TOTAL:	

NOTES/ACCOMPLISHMENTS

DAY 35 – Date_____

	FOOD ITEM	TOTAL SUGAR CALORIES
MEAL 1		
SNACK		
MEAL 2		
SNACK		
MEAL 3		
SNACK		
	TOTAL:	

NOTES/ACCOMPLISHMENTS

This page intentionally left blank

WEEKLY MEAL PLANNER
Week of _____

	BREAKFAST	LUNCH	DINNER	SNACKS
MON				
TUE				
WED				
THU				
FRI				
SAT				
SUN				

DAY 36 – Date_____

	FOOD ITEM	TOTAL SUGAR CALORIES
MEAL 1		
SNACK		
MEAL 2		
SNACK		
MEAL 3		
SNACK		
	TOTAL:	

NOTES/ACCOMPLISHMENTS

_____
_____
_____

DAY 37 – Date_____

	FOOD ITEM	TOTAL SUGAR CALORIES
MEAL 1		
SNACK		
MEAL 2		
SNACK		
MEAL 3		
SNACK		
	TOTAL:	

NOTES/ACCOMPLISHMENTS

DAY 38 – Date_____

	FOOD ITEM	TOTAL SUGAR CALORIES
MEAL 1		
SNACK		
MEAL 2		
SNACK		
MEAL 3		
SNACK		
	TOTAL:	

NOTES/ACCOMPLISHMENTS

DAY 39 – Date_____

	FOOD ITEM	TOTAL SUGAR CALORIES
MEAL 1		
SNACK		
MEAL 2		
SNACK		
MEAL 3		
SNACK		
	TOTAL:	

NOTES/ACCOMPLISHMENTS

DAY 40 – Date_____

	FOOD ITEM	TOTAL SUGAR CALORIES
MEAL 1		
SNACK		
MEAL 2		
SNACK		
MEAL 3		
SNACK		
	TOTAL:	

NOTES/ACCOMPLISHMENTS

DAY 41 – Date_____

	FOOD ITEM	TOTAL SUGAR CALORIES
MEAL 1		
SNACK		
MEAL 2		
SNACK		
MEAL 3		
SNACK		
	TOTAL:	

NOTES/ACCOMPLISHMENTS

DAY 42 – Date_____

	FOOD ITEM	TOTAL SUGAR CALORIES
MEAL 1		
SNACK		
MEAL 2		
SNACK		
MEAL 3		
SNACK		
	TOTAL:	

NOTES/ACCOMPLISHMENTS

_____
_____
_____

WEEKLY MEAL PLANNER
Week of _____

	BREAKFAST	LUNCH	DINNER	SNACKS
MON				
TUE				
WED				
THU				
FRI				
SAT				
SUN				

DAY 43 – Date_____

	FOOD ITEM	TOTAL SUGAR CALORIES
MEAL 1		
SNACK		
MEAL 2		
SNACK		
MEAL 3		
SNACK		
	TOTAL:	

NOTES/ACCOMPLISHMENTS

DAY 44 – Date_____

	FOOD ITEM	TOTAL SUGAR CALORIES
MEAL 1		
SNACK		
MEAL 2		
SNACK		
MEAL 3		
SNACK		
	TOTAL:	

NOTES/ACCOMPLISHMENTS

DAY 45 – Date_____

	FOOD ITEM	TOTAL SUGAR CALORIES
MEAL 1		
SNACK		
MEAL 2		
SNACK		
MEAL 3		
SNACK		
	TOTAL:	

NOTES/ACCOMPLISHMENTS

DAY 46 – Date_____

	FOOD ITEM	TOTAL SUGAR CALORIES
MEAL 1		
SNACK		
MEAL 2		
SNACK		
MEAL 3		
SNACK		
	TOTAL:	

NOTES/ACCOMPLISHMENTS

DAY 47 – Date_____

	FOOD ITEM	TOTAL SUGAR CALORIES
MEAL 1		
SNACK		
MEAL 2		
SNACK		
MEAL 3		
SNACK		
	TOTAL:	

NOTES/ACCOMPLISHMENTS

DAY 48 – Date_____

	FOOD ITEM	TOTAL SUGAR CALORIES
MEAL 1		
SNACK		
MEAL 2		
SNACK		
MEAL 3		
SNACK		
	TOTAL:	

NOTES/ACCOMPLISHMENTS

DAY 49 – Date_____

	FOOD ITEM	TOTAL SUGAR CALORIES
MEAL 1		
SNACK		
MEAL 2		
SNACK		
MEAL 3		
SNACK		
	TOTAL:	

NOTES/ACCOMPLISHMENTS

WEEKLY MEAL PLANNER
Week of _____

	BREAKFAST	LUNCH	DINNER	SNACKS
MON				
TUE				
WED				
THU				
FRI				
SAT				
SUN				

DAY 50 – Date_____

	FOOD ITEM	TOTAL SUGAR CALORIES
MEAL 1		
SNACK		
MEAL 2		
SNACK		
MEAL 3		
SNACK		
	TOTAL:	

NOTES/ACCOMPLISHMENTS

DAY 51 – Date_____

	FOOD ITEM	TOTAL SUGAR CALORIES
MEAL 1		
SNACK		
MEAL 2		
SNACK		
MEAL 3		
SNACK		
	TOTAL:	

NOTES/ACCOMPLISHMENTS

DAY 52 – Date_____

	FOOD ITEM	TOTAL SUGAR CALORIES
MEAL 1		
SNACK		
MEAL 2		
SNACK		
MEAL 3		
SNACK		
	TOTAL:	

NOTES/ACCOMPLISHMENTS

DAY 53 – Date_____

	FOOD ITEM	TOTAL SUGAR CALORIES
MEAL 1		
SNACK		
MEAL 2		
SNACK		
MEAL 3		
SNACK		
	TOTAL:	

NOTES/ACCOMPLISHMENTS

DAY 54 – Date_____

	FOOD ITEM	TOTAL SUGAR CALORIES
MEAL 1		
SNACK		
MEAL 2		
SNACK		
MEAL 3		
SNACK		
	TOTAL:	

NOTES/ACCOMPLISHMENTS

DAY 55 – Date_____

	FOOD ITEM	TOTAL SUGAR CALORIES
MEAL 1		
SNACK		
MEAL 2		
SNACK		
MEAL 3		
SNACK		
	TOTAL:	

NOTES/ACCOMPLISHMENTS

_____
_____
_____

DAY 56 – Date_____

	FOOD ITEM	TOTAL SUGAR CALORIES
MEAL 1		
SNACK		
MEAL 2		
SNACK		
MEAL 3		
SNACK		
	TOTAL:	

NOTES/ACCOMPLISHMENTS

Week of _____

	BREAKFAST	LUNCH	DINNER	SNACKS
MON				
TUE				
WED				
THU				
FRI				
SAT				
SUN				

DAY 57 – Date_____

	FOOD ITEM	TOTAL SUGAR CALORIES
MEAL 1		
SNACK		
MEAL 2		
SNACK		
MEAL 3		
SNACK		
	TOTAL:	

NOTES/ACCOMPLISHMENTS

DAY 58 – Date_____

	FOOD ITEM	TOTAL SUGAR CALORIES
MEAL 1		
SNACK		
MEAL 2		
SNACK		
MEAL 3		
SNACK		
	TOTAL:	

NOTES/ACCOMPLISHMENTS

DAY 59 – Date_____

	FOOD ITEM	TOTAL SUGAR CALORIES
MEAL 1		
SNACK		
MEAL 2		
SNACK		
MEAL 3		
SNACK		
	TOTAL:	

NOTES/ACCOMPLISHMENTS

DAY 60 – Date_____

	FOOD ITEM	TOTAL SUGAR CALORIES
MEAL 1		
SNACK		
MEAL 2		
SNACK		
MEAL 3		
SNACK		
	TOTAL:	

NOTES/ACCOMPLISHMENTS

AFTER PICTURE

MY WEIGHT_____

WHAT I'M THINKING/HOW I FEEL: _____

_____

_____

_____

_____

_____

_____

FAVORITE RECIPES

Recipe Name: _____
*Serves:*_____

Oven Temp_____Prep Time_____Cook Time _____

Ingredients:

Preparation Directions:

Cooking Directions:

Notes:

FAVORITE RECIPES

Recipe Name: _____
*Serves:*_____

Oven Temp_____Prep Time_____Cook Time _____

Ingredients:

Preparation Directions:

Cooking Directions:

Notes:

FAVORITE RECIPES

Recipe Name: _____
*Serves:*_____

Oven Temp_____Prep Time_____Cook Time _____

Ingredients:

_____   _____

_____   _____

_____   _____

_____   _____

Preparation Directions:

_____
_____
_____
_____
_____

Cooking Directions:

_____
_____
_____
_____
_____

Notes:

_____
_____
_____
_____
_____

FAVORITE RECIPES

Recipe Name: _____
Serves:_____

Oven Temp_____Prep Time_____Cook Time _____

Ingredients:

_____   _____

_____   _____

_____   _____

_____   _____

Preparation Directions:
_____
_____
_____
_____
_____

Cooking Directions:
_____
_____
_____
_____
_____

Notes:
_____
_____
_____
_____
_____

FAVORITE RECIPES

Recipe Name: _____
*Serves:*_____

Oven Temp_____Prep Time_____Cook Time _____

Ingredients:

Preparation Directions:

Cooking Directions:

Notes:

FAVORITE RECIPES

Recipe Name: _____
*Serves:*_____

Oven Temp_____Prep Time_____Cook Time _____

Ingredients:
_____ _____
_____ _____
_____ _____
_____ _____

Preparation Directions:
_____
_____
_____
_____
_____

Cooking Directions:
_____
_____
_____
_____
_____

Notes:
_____
_____
_____
_____
_____

FAVORITE RECIPES

Recipe Name: _____
*Serves:*_____

Oven Temp_____Prep Time_____Cook Time _____

Ingredients:

_____   _____

_____   _____

_____   _____

_____   _____

Preparation Directions:

_____
_____
_____
_____
_____

Cooking Directions:

_____
_____
_____
_____
_____

Notes:

_____
_____
_____
_____
_____

FAVORITE RECIPES

Recipe Name: _____
Serves:_____

Oven Temp_____Prep Time_____Cook Time _____

Ingredients:
_____   _____
_____   _____
_____   _____
_____   _____

Preparation Directions:
_____
_____
_____
_____
_____

Cooking Directions:
_____
_____
_____
_____
_____

Notes:
_____
_____
_____
_____
_____

NOTES

NOTES

NOTES

NOTES

SHOPPING LIST

SHOPPING LIST

SHOPPING LIST

Made in the USA
San Bernardino, CA
19 February 2015